SIMPLIFIED GUIDE ON

ESSENTIAL OIL FOR EMOTIONAL RESILIENCE

Unlock The Power Of Aromatherapy To Navigate Life's Challenges, Stimulate Olfactory System + More - A Practical book For Emotional Balance

DR. ARIYA REYNA

CONTENTS

Copyright © 2023, By Dr. Ariya Reyna

All Rights Reserved

This book is protected by copyright law, and any unauthorized reproduction, distribution, or transmission of the contents, in whole or in part, without the prior written consent of the author and the publisher is prohibited.

DISCLIAMER

This book is intended for informational purposes only and is not a substitute for professional medical advice, diagnosis, or treatment. The information provided in this book is based on the author's research and personal experiences and is not meant to replace the advice of healthcare professionals.

Readers are encouraged to consult with their healthcare providers before beginning any new exercise, wellness, or health program.

The author and publisher of this book are not responsible for any specific health or allergy needs that may require medical supervision and are not liable for any damages or negative consequences from any treatment, action, application, or preparation, to any person reading or following the information in this book.

The content of this book is not intended to be a substitute for professional medical advice, diagnosis, or treatment. Always seek the advice of your physician or other qualified health provider with any questions you may have regarding a medical condition.

The author and publisher disclaim responsibility for any adverse effects that may result from the use or application of the information contained in this book.

References to specific products, services, or organizations do not imply endorsement or recommendation by the author or the publisher.

The inclusion of such references is for illustrative purposes only. Thank you for reading and respecting the terms outlined in this disclaimer.

CHAPTER ONE

Introduction

Emotional resilience is an important part of total well-being since it encompasses our ability to adapt to and recover from life's obstacles. Many people are turning to holistic techniques to achieve emotional balance, with essential oils emerging as a popular alternative. Essential oils, which are produced from plants, have medicinal characteristics that can have a favorable influence on our moods. This article delves into the notion of emotional resilience, the function of essential oils in developing emotional well-being, the selection criteria for essential oils, and several strategies for using them to improve emotional health.

Recognizing Emotional Resilience

The ability to cope with and overcome hardship, stress, and life's uncertainties is referred to as emotional resilience. Adapting to change, preserving mental well-being, and rebounding from setbacks are all part of it. In essence, emotional resilience is the psychological strength that allows people to face life's adversities with a positive attitude.

Emotional resilience is influenced by a variety of elements, including one's mentality, coping methods, social support, and self-awareness. Self-reflection, learning from experiences, and building a proactive attitude toward obstacles are all part of the process of developing emotional resilience.

When people confront emotional problems, their nervous systems might respond with increased stress, prompting a variety of emotional responses. This is where essential oils may help, providing a natural and comprehensive approach to mental well-being.

Essential Oils' Impact On Emotional Well-Being

Essential oils have been used in traditional medicine and aromatherapy for millennia for their medicinal benefits on the body and mind. Essential oils may be great friends when it comes to emotional well-being.

The olfactory system, which is responsible for our sense of smell, is closely linked to the limbic system of the brain, which regulates emotions and memories. As a result, inhaling essential oil aromas can have a direct effect on our mental state.

Certain essential oils have been shown to enhance relaxation, reduce tension, and improve mood. Lavender oil, for example, is known for its relaxing characteristics, whilst citrus scents like bergamot and orange may be uplifting and stimulating. With its earthy and calming aroma, frankincense is frequently used to create emotional equilibrium.

Furthermore, essential oils may be an effective tool for dealing with various emotions. Chamomile and ylang-ylang, for example, may help ease anxiety, whilst peppermint and eucalyptus may give a refreshing and stimulating boost to counteract exhaustion.

Selecting The Best Essential Oils

Individual tastes, distinct emotional demands, and intended results must all be considered when choosing the best essential oils for emotional support. To ensure their efficiency and safety, essential oils must be of high quality and pure.

1. Lavender (Lavandula angustifolia): Lavender is a versatile oil with relaxing effects that can help relieve tension and promote relaxation.

2. Bergamot (Citrus bergamia): Bergamot's zesty and uplifting scent helps improve mood and reduce anxiety.

3. Frankincense (Boswellia carterii): This earthy oil is frequently used for anchoring and fostering emotional equilibrium.

4. Chamomile (Matricaria chamomilla): Chamomile has calming effects and is widely used to relieve stress and promote relaxation.

5. Cananga odorata (Ylang-Ylang): Known for its flowery and sweet aroma, ylang-ylang can help relieve tension and anxiety while fostering relaxation.

6. Peppermint (Mentha piperita): Refreshing and energizing, peppermint oil can deliver an immediate energy boost while also combating weariness.

It is critical to consider personal preferences as well as any potential sensitivities or allergies when including essential oils in an emotional resilience regimen. Experimenting with different oils and mixes might help people find which ones best match their emotional requirements.

Methods Of Emotional Support Application

Essential oils may be used in a variety of ways to achieve emotional effects. The approach selected is frequently determined by personal preferences and the unique emotional difficulties being addressed.

1. Diffusion: Using an essential oil diffuser disperses aromatic molecules into the air, making them available for inhalation. This strategy is useful for establishing emotional equilibrium by producing a tranquil or uplifting ambiance in a room.

2. Topical Application: Applying essential oils to the skin after diluting them with carrier oil enables absorption through the pores. Wrists, temples, and the back of the neck are common application sites. This strategy is appropriate for providing targeted emotional assistance.

3. Inhalation: Inhaling essential oils directly from the bottle or by dabbing a few drops on a tissue is a quick and easy approach to feel their benefits. This strategy is especially useful for providing emotional support when on the road.

4. Baths: A few drops of essential oils added to a warm bath produce a relaxing and pleasant experience. This strategy is perfect for unwinding and relaxing after a long day.

It is vital to note that essential oils are very concentrated, and correct dilution is critical, especially for topical use. Additionally, before introducing essential oils into a wellness program, anyone with pre-existing medical issues or pregnant women should check with a healthcare provider.

Conclusion

The use of essential oils provides a natural and comprehensive approach to supporting emotional well-being in the development of emotional resilience. Individuals can use essential oils to induce relaxation, reduce stress, and raise mood by understanding emotional resilience as the capacity to handle life's adversities with a positive mentality.

Choosing the proper essential oils requires taking into account personal tastes as well as specific emotional demands, and application techniques differ to meet individual preferences and circumstances. Incorporating essential oils into a health regimen, whether through diffusion, topical application, inhalation, or baths, can help to increase emotional resilience and maintain a balanced and pleasant emotional state.

As people seek holistic methods to emotional well-being, essential oils stand out as a powerful and adaptable tool, providing not just fragrant pleasures but also a road to emotional balance.

CHAPTER TWO

Essential Oil Blending For Emotional Resilience

For ages, essential oils have been utilized to improve mental well-being and resilience. Strategically combining these oils can increase their particular characteristics, resulting in potent mixtures that assist emotional wellness. The synergy of essential oil mixtures can be very useful for emotional resilience.

Understanding the characteristics of various oils is critical when creating a combination for emotional resilience. Some essential oils are recognized for their relaxing properties, while others are known for their uplifting or grounding properties. Lavender, for example, is known for its relaxing characteristics, bergamot for its energizing capabilities, and frankincense for its grounding and centering virtues.

A typical blend for emotional resilience may contain lavender, bergamot, and frankincense. The relaxing effect of lavender helps to relieve tension and anxiety, while bergamot delivers a surge of optimism and frankincense provides a sense of stability. These oils combine to provide a balanced combination that promotes emotional strength and resilience.

It is critical to examine the ratios while combining essential oils. To generate a well-rounded scent and therapeutic effect, a base note, a middle note, and a top note should be used. In the instance of emotional resilience, the base note can be frankincense, the middle note can be bergamot, and the top note can be lavender.

When crafting blends, experimentation is essential. Begin with a small quantity of each oil and alter the ratios to your liking. It's crucial to remember that individual reactions to fragrances might differ, so it's best to start slowly and gradually increase the concentration.

Once created, the mix can be diffused using an essential oil diffuser or used topically after being diluted with a carrier oil. The therapeutic benefits of the oils may be absorbed by inhaling the scent of the mix or applying it to pulse points, boosting emotional balance and resilience.

Emotional Balance And Aromatherapy

Aromatherapy, or the therapeutic application of essential oils, is a potent technique for improving emotional equilibrium. The olfactory system, which is responsible for scent, is intimately related to the limbic system of the brain, which is involved in emotions, memories, and arousal. Because of this link, aromatherapy is a direct and powerful technique to alter mood and emotional well-being.

To get the benefits of aromatherapy for emotional balance, essential oils with specific qualities must be used. Popular oils for relaxation and stress reduction include lavender, chamomile, and ylang-ylang. These oils have relaxing effects on the neurological system, which helps to relieve stress and produce a sense of peace.

Citrus oils, on the other hand, such as lemon, orange, and grapefruit, are wonderful for boosting energy and mood. Their bright and cheerful smells may elevate one's mood and create a happy environment. Combining oils from different categories, such as relaxing and uplifting oils, can result in a well-rounded combination that addresses different areas of emotional balance.

Aromatherapy may be incorporated into everyday activities in a variety of ways. Diffusers, which disseminate essential oil molecules into the air, are a popular and convenient option. A few drops of the chosen essential oil or combination added to a diffuser may create a relaxing and healing environment.

Making personal inhalers or applying diluted essential oils to pulse points, on the other hand, enables on-the-go usage. Throughout the day, inhaling the scent of the oils gives constant support for emotional equilibrium.

Aromatherapy may also be included in self-care routines, such as adding a few drops of essential oil to a warm bath or combining essential oils with carrier oils for a relaxing massage. Aromatherapy's sensory experience enriches these activities, making them more pleasurable and adding to overall emotional well-being.

Essential Oils For Stress Reduction

Stress is an unavoidable aspect of life, yet good stress management is critical for general well-being. Essential oils provide a natural and comprehensive approach to stress management, addressing both the physical and emotional elements of the condition.

With its relaxing and soothing characteristics, lavender oil is a well-known stress reliever. Inhaling the lavender smell or putting it to pulse points might help induce relaxation and relieve stress. Furthermore, because of their relaxing effects on the neurological system, chamomile and rose essential oils are good alternatives for stress management.

Citrus oils, such as bergamot and orange, are effective stress relievers. Their uplifting and revitalizing smells can help improve one's mood and alleviate exhaustion and worry. These oils work especially well when diffused or put on personal inhalers for quick and easy usage during stressful times.

Frankincense, with its grounding and centering characteristics, is another effective stress-relieving oil. Inhaling the perfume of frankincense or diluting it with a carrier oil and applying it to the skin helps relax the mind and body.

Creating a combination of these stress-relieving oils can boost their efficacy. For example, a basic combination of lavender, bergamot, and frankincense can give a well-rounded approach to stress management. For a more tailored and focused experience, diffuse this combination at home or apply it topically.

While essential oils can help with stress management, they should only be used as part of a complete approach to well-being. Healthy lifestyle choices such as frequent exercise, a balanced diet, and proper sleep are also important in stress management and reduction.

Aromatic Oils Can Help You Relax.

Relaxation is an important part of sustaining emotional resiliency. Aromatic oils, which are obtained from diverse plant sources, are a natural and delightful approach to promote relaxation and create a quiet environment.

Lavender, known for its relaxing characteristics, is a popular oil for encouraging relaxation. Its calming aroma can aid in the reduction of tension and stress, making it an excellent choice for relaxation mixes. Combining lavender with other soothing oils, such as chamomile or geranium, can boost its relaxing properties.

Chamomile essential oil, especially Roman chamomile, is another good option for encouraging relaxation. Its delicate and flowery perfume has a relaxing effect on the neurological system, making it ideal for crafting mixes that promote relaxation and tranquillity.

With its sweet and exotic aroma, ylang-ylang is recognized for its ability to encourage relaxation and alleviate stress. When ylang-ylang is added to relaxation blends, it offers a sensuous and relaxing quality, making it a popular option for generating a peaceful atmosphere.

Massage mixtures are a diverse technique to encourage relaxation using scented oils. Diluting essential oils with a carrier oil and massaging them into the skin not only enables skin absorption but also improves the sensory experience. To make a wonderful massage blend, combine oils like lavender, chamomile, and ylang-ylang with a carrier oil like sweet almond or jojoba oil.

Aromatic oils, in addition to massage, can be utilized in other relaxation-inducing activities such as meditation and bath rituals. Adding a few drops of essential oil to a warm bath at home produces a spa-like experience that promotes relaxation and relieves stress.

To summarize, using essential oils for emotional resilience requires careful mixing, understanding the qualities of particular oils, and incorporating aromatherapy into everyday activities. The flexibility of essential oils makes them useful tools for boosting general emotional well-being, whether it's making a blend for emotional strength, employing aromatherapy for emotional balance, managing stress with particular oils, or inducing relaxation with aromatic oils.

CHAPTER THREE

Essential Oils For Emotional Resilience That Are Uplifting And Energizing

Maintaining emotional resilience is critical for general well-being in today's fast-paced society. Essential oils have long been utilized for their medicinal effects, including their ability to elevate and stimulate the mind and body. Adding uplifting and invigorating essential oils to your daily routine may be a valuable tool for boosting emotional resilience.

1. Citrus oils, such as lemon, orange, and grapefruit, are well known for their energizing and uplifting effects. Citrus oils' bright and zesty scent can help relieve tension and exhaustion while also encouraging a cheerful and invigorated mentality. Diffusing these oils or putting a few drops into a personal inhaler is a quick and easy method to get their mood-boosting effects.

2. Peppermint: The aroma of peppermint essential oil is both invigorating and stimulating. Inhaling peppermint oil helps improve alertness and focus, making it a great alternative for dealing with mental exhaustion. Furthermore, peppermint oil contains cooling effects that can help with clarity and focus, making it a popular choice for individuals looking for an energy boost.

3. Eucalyptus: Although eucalyptus essential oil is commonly linked with respiratory benefits, its energizing scent can also assist with mental well-being. Inhaling eucalyptus oil may generate a sensation of vigor and openness, making it an excellent addition to mixes intended to elevate the spirits. Consider diffusing eucalyptus oil to enjoy its energizing benefits during times of stress or low energy.

4. Rosemary essential oil is well-known for its invigorating and purifying qualities. Inhaling rosemary's scent can assist in boosting focus and memory, making it an excellent choice for people

suffering from mental tiredness or problems. In a diffuser combination, combining rosemary and citrus oils can have a synergistic impact, improving the overall uplifting experience.

5. Bergamot essential oil has a pleasant zesty scent with floral overtones and is obtained from the peel of the bergamot orange. It is well-known for its relaxing and mood-balancing properties. Bergamot oil can help elevate emotions and produce a sense of joy, making it an effective tool for stress management and emotional resilience.

There are several ways to include these uplifting and energetic essential oils in your everyday routine. Diffusing essential oils at your home or office, adding a few drops to a warm bath, or making a personal inhaler to take with you throughout the day are all excellent ways to reap their mood-boosting effects. Experiment with numerous oil blends to find the one that best suits your tastes and emotional requirements.

Anxiety And Mood Swings Essential Oils

Anxiety and mood swings are widespread problems in our contemporary lives, and finding natural solutions to these problems is critical for emotional resilience. Essential oils, with their powerful aromatic components, can help to promote emotional balance and stability. The following essential oils are well-known for their soothing and mood-regulating properties:

1. Lavender essential oil is well-known for its soothing and relaxing properties. The calming perfume of lavender can help relieve anxiety and produce a sense of calm. Lavender oil is a flexible and soothing alternative for controlling stress and increasing mental well-being, whether diffused in the air, used topically (diluted with a carrier oil), or added to a warm bath.

2. Chamomile: Chamomile essential oil is recognized for its anti-anxiety qualities and is extracted from the chamomile flower.

Chamomile's pleasant and vegetal aroma might aid in soothing the nervous system and relieve tension. Incorporating chamomile oil into your sleep ritual or diffusing it during stressful times might help you feel more peaceful and centered.

3. Ylang-Ylang: With its rich and flowery perfume, ylang-ylang essential oil is frequently used to produce emotions of joy and relaxation. This oil is well-known for its ability to regulate emotions and alleviate uneasiness. Diffusing ylang-ylang oil or incorporating a few drops into a massage oil is a great approach to get its mood-stabilizing effects.

4. Frankincense essential oil provides a grounding and balancing influence on the psyche. It is frequently used to achieve emotional balance and tranquility. Inhaling the scent of frankincense or using it physically can help reduce anxiety and promote emotional well-being.

5. Patchouli essential oil is noted for its relaxing and grounding effects due to its earthy and sweet

fragrance. It can be especially effective for people who suffer from mood swings or mental instability. Diffusing patchouli oil or mixing it with carrier oil for topical application can aid in the creation of a calming and pleasant environment.

It's critical to tailor your strategy when utilizing essential oils for anxiety and mood swings. Experiment with different oils and application methods to see what works best for you. Whether you like diffusing essential oils around your house, applying them to pulse points, or incorporating them into self-care routines, the key to reaping the cumulative effects of these natural therapies is persistence.

Daily Practices For Emotional Resilience

Developing emotional resilience entails developing habits and behaviors that promote mental and emotional well-being. While essential oils might help with this, adopting other daily habits can boost your overall resilience. Here are some essential ways to increase emotional resilience in your everyday life:

1. Mindfulness Meditation: You may increase your awareness of your thoughts and feelings by practicing mindfulness meditation. This technique promotes nonjudgmental observation of the present moment, which fosters emotional resilience by decreasing response to stimuli. Consider beginning your day with a short mindfulness meditation to create a good tone.

2. Keeping a thankfulness notebook is an effective strategy for fostering a good outlook. Take a few moments each day to focus on and write down things you are grateful for. This technique directs your attention to the good parts of your life, promoting resilience in the face of adversity.

3. Regular physical activity has been related to increased mood and resilience. Exercise releases endorphins, the body's natural mood elevators, and serves as a healthy stress release.

Including movement in your routine, whether it's a quick stroll, a yoga session, or a complete exercise, can have a great influence on your mental well-being.

4. Healthy Sleep Habits: Sleeping well is critical for emotional resiliency. Setting a consistent sleep schedule, maintaining a pleasant sleep environment, and practicing relaxation methods before bedtime can all help you sleep better. A calm mind is better equipped to handle the challenges of life.

5. Social Connection: Developing meaningful connections with people is a critical component of emotional resilience. Having a support network, whether via family, friends, or community activity, gives emotional support during stressful times. Maintain open contact with individuals you trust and make time for social activities.

6. Self-Compassion: Practicing self-compassion is treating yourself with care and understanding, particularly during difficult times. Recognize your

feelings without judgment and treat yourself as you would a friend. This method promotes resilience by encouraging a positive and supportive inner conversation.

7. Engaging in creative endeavors, such as painting, music, or writing, can be a therapeutic outlet for feelings. Creative expression enables self-reflection and can act as a helpful coping tool during stressful times.

8. Digital Detox: Emotional well-being must limit exposure to continual digital stimuli. Set limits on screen use, especially before bedtime, and include disconnecting moments to allow for mental and emotional recharge.

When these everyday routines are combined with the use of uplifting essential oils, a comprehensive approach to emotional resilience is created. Each component strengthens the others, resulting in a solid foundation for managing life's ups and downs with grace and strength.

CHAPTER FOUR

Essential Oil Safety Considerations And Precautions

While essential oils provide a natural and comprehensive approach to emotional well-being, they must be used with caution and understanding. When using essential oils in your regimen, keep the following safety considerations and precautions in mind:

1. Dilution: Because essential oils are very concentrated and strong, using them directly on the skin without dilution might cause irritation or sensitivity. Before using essential oils topically, always dilute them with a carrier oil, such as jojoba or sweet almond oil. For people, 1-2 drops of essential oil per teaspoon of carrier oil is a good starting point.

2. Skin Sensitivity: Different people may react differently to essential oils. Before using the essential oil on a large scale, do a patch test by

applying a diluted solution to a small area of the skin and watching for any adverse effects. Certain oils, such as citrus oils, might make you more sensitive to sunlight, so use caution when applying them to exposed skin before going outside.

3. Pregnancy and Children: Essential oils may cause sensitivity in pregnant women and young children, and some oils are contraindicated during pregnancy. Before using essential oils during pregnancy or on children, it is best to speak with a healthcare practitioner. Use particular caution with infants and young children and use oils that are usually recognized as safe for their age range.

4. Quality Is Important: The quality of essential oils might vary, so it's critical to select high-quality, pure oils from recognized suppliers. Look for oils branded "100% pure" and subjected to third-party testing for quality and purity. Synthetic fragrance oils should be avoided since they lack the therapeutic properties of genuine essential oils.

5. Allergies and Sensitivities: If you have known allergies or sensitivities to certain plants or chemicals, use essential oils produced from those sources with caution.

Be mindful of cross-allergens and, if in doubt, seek the advice of an allergist or a healthcare expert before using essential oils.

6. Internal Use: While some essential oils are classified as food-grade, using them internally without sufficient expertise and advice is not advised. Essential oils can have negative side effects and may interfere with pharmaceuticals. Before contemplating internal usage, consult with a competent aromatherapist or healthcare practitioner.

7. Storage: Essential oils are light, heat, and air-sensitive, which can impair their quality over time. To keep essential oils potent, store them in dark glass bottles in a cold, dark environment.

Keep undiluted oils out of the reach of children and exercise caution while handling them.

8. Consultation with Healthcare Professionals: If you have underlying health issues, are on medications, or have questions regarding the appropriateness of certain essential oils for your circumstances, it is best to consult with a healthcare expert or experienced aromatherapist. They may provide you with specialized advice based on your specific health requirements.

To summarize, while essential oils can be useful tools for emotional resilience, they should be used with caution and consideration for individual variances.

You may reap the advantages of these strong plant extracts while also establishing a safe and supportive atmosphere for emotional well-being if you follow safety precautions and incorporate them into a holistic health regimen.

A Therapeutic Journey With Essential Oils For Emotional Resilience

1. Personalized Essential Oil Rituals

Personalized essential oil rituals have emerged as important strategies for promoting resilience in the field of emotional well-being. The idea is to adjust essential oil use to individual tastes, requirements, and emotional states. Essential oils, with their different olfactory qualities, may be used to construct individualized rituals that encourage emotional balance and resilience.

Self-awareness is the first step in creating individualized essential oil routines. Individuals go on a journey to uncover emotional triggers, stresses, and places in need of assistance. This insight serves as the foundation for choosing essential oils that correspond to one's emotional requirements. Lavender and chamomile, for example, may be used to calm, but citrus oils like bergamot or orange can be used to elevate and revitalize.

Creating a tailored essential oil ritual entails selecting the appropriate application method. Common methods include diffusing oils in the home, using them topically, and incorporating them into bath routines. The goal is to effortlessly incorporate these rituals into daily life, making them a natural part of the individual's routine.

Furthermore, the timing of these ceremonies is critical. Morning rituals may include exhilarating odors to get the day started, while nighttime routines may include relaxing aromas to unwind. The importance of consistency cannot be overstated, and adding essential oils into daily routines enhances their therapeutic benefits over time.

The versatility of individual essential oil routines is what makes them so appealing. As emotional requirements change, so should the oils and rituals. Individuals may adapt to life's swings with a specific emotional support system using this dynamic technique. During times of high stress, for example, a specific blend of soothing oils might be diffused, or a relaxing bath practice can be implemented.

In essence, individualized essential oil rituals are about building a deep connection with oneself and using essential oils' inherent therapeutic capabilities to manage the intricacies of emotions.

2. Using Essential Oils For Self-Care

Self-care is a critical component of emotional resilience, and essential oils play an important role in this holistic approach. The use of essential oils in self-care routines increases their effectiveness, providing individuals with a practical and fun approach to prioritizing their emotional well-being.

One of the most significant advantages of adding essential oils into self-care is its capacity to improve relaxation and stress alleviation. Aromatherapy, which uses essential oils to enhance psychological and physical well-being, has emerged as a powerful tool in self-care practices. Diffusing calming smells like lavender or chamomile during meditation or yoga sessions generates a peaceful environment that promotes deeper relaxation.

The use of essential oils topically in self-care rituals such as massage or skincare regimens provides another layer of therapeutic benefit. Massage using oils like eucalyptus or peppermint can relieve stress and produce a sense of refreshment. Additionally, selecting oils with skincare benefits improves both the physical and mental elements of self-care.

Essential oils serve as anchors in the self-care journey in the context of emotional resilience. Aromas are potent triggers for pleasant emotional states due to the olfactory system's direct relationship to the brain's emotional center. Individuals can establish a good mentality and increase emotional resilience over time by integrating smells that connect with sentiments of pleasure, calm, or thankfulness.

The flexibility of essential oils enables a wide range of self-care applications. The possibilities range from crafting unique scents that conjure happy memories to incorporating them into everyday beauty practices. The goal is to make these activities purposeful, transforming everyday moments of self-care into chances for emotional sustenance.

To summarize, including essential oils in self-care activities is a conscious and pleasurable strategy to boost emotional resilience. Individuals can achieve a healthy balance that enhances their emotional well-being by combining the sensory enjoyment of scents with focused self-care activities.

3. Case Studies: Real-Life Examples

Real-world uses of essential oils in the promotion of emotional resilience demonstrate the significant influence of these natural therapies on people's lives. Case studies show how tailored essential oil rituals and their incorporation into self-care routines have transformed into transformational tools for regulating emotions and building resilience.

Consider Sarah, a young worker who suffers from chronic stress and anxiety. Sarah discovered lavender and frankincense essential oils that spoke to her through a tailored approach. She integrated these oils into her regular regimen by diffusing them during the day and applying a diluted combination to pulse points before bed. Sarah reported a considerable reduction in stress levels and increased sleep quality after a few weeks, illustrating the usefulness of individualized essential oil routines.

In another case, Mark, a middle-aged man experiencing spells of depression, investigated the use of essential oils in his self-care regimen. He introduced citrus oils such as orange and grapefruit into his daily practice, diffusing them while meditating. The stimulating smells not only revived him in the mornings but also contributed to a more optimistic attitude throughout the day. Mark's story demonstrates the power of mindful essential oil use in creating emotional resilience.

These case studies highlight the uniqueness of essential oil uses. What works for one individual may not work for another, highlighting the necessity of self-discovery on the path to emotional well-being. Because essential oils are adaptable, they allow for experimentation until the correct blend is found, making it a dynamic and changing process.

An increasing body of research supports essential oils' usefulness in fostering emotional resilience as more people share their experiences with them. These real-world applications provide promise to individuals looking for natural and comprehensive methods for emotional well-being.

4. Future Emotional Wellness And Essential Oil Trends

Essential oils will continue to be integrated into mainstream practices in the future of emotional well-being, driven by growing trends and scientific discoveries. Essential oils are anticipated to play an increasingly important part in holistic approaches to emotional well-being as an understanding of the mind-body link grows.

The combination of technology and aromatherapy is one rising trend. Smart diffusers, which include programmable capabilities and can be operated via mobile applications, are becoming increasingly popular. This marriage of technology and essential oils enables accurate and customized dispersion that caters to individual tastes and emotional requirements. Diffuser sessions may be scheduled, with different oils being blended at specified times to produce individualized aromatherapy experiences.

Furthermore, scientific study on essential oils' psychological and physiological benefits is developing. More focused and evidence-based uses are expected to develop as our understanding of the medicinal characteristics of various oils deepens. This research might lead to the creation of tailored essential oil blends for certain emotional difficulties, improving their usefulness even more.

Personalized essential oil compositions based on genetic and biomarker data are potentially possible in the future. Individuals may have access to specific essential oil suggestions that fit with their particular genetic predispositions and emotional profiles as the area of personalized medicine improves. This level of formulation expertise may enhance the therapeutic advantages of essential oils for emotional resilience.

Environmental concerns are also impacting the essential oil business. Essential oils supplied sustainably and ethically are gaining popularity as customers become more concerned about the environmental effects of their decisions. Future trends may see a greater emphasis on eco-friendly procedures in essential oil production, ensuring that the whole process, from cultivation to extraction, adheres to environmental stewardship standards.

Finally, the future of emotional wellness and essential oils will be defined by a harmonic combination of old knowledge, current technology, and scientific advances.

Essential oils are positioned to remain a cornerstone of holistic approaches to emotional resilience as our awareness of the deep relationship between emotions and well-being grows, with advancements and research opening the way for ever more individualized and effective therapies.

Conclusion On Essential Oil For Emotional Resilience

Finally, essential oils appear as effective allies in promoting emotional resilience. These oils, with their aromatic components and medicinal characteristics, play an important role in establishing a balanced and resilient mental state. Individuals have a tailored toolset for managing stress, anxiety, and other emotional difficulties thanks to the varied spectrum of essential oils, each with its distinct aroma and therapeutic advantages.

Certain essential oils, such as lavender, chamomile, and bergamot, have been shown in studies to improve mood and reduce symptoms of emotional distress.

The fragrances of these oils, whether diffused, applied topically, or breathed, have the capacity to elicit soothing reactions in the brain, affecting emotions and stress levels. Furthermore, the ritualistic use of essential oils in self-care routines promotes awareness and relaxation, which improves emotional well-being.

While essential oils are not a cure-all, they do contribute significantly to holistic approaches to emotional resilience. Their natural roots connect with modern wellness desires, providing individuals with a natural and complementary approach to improving mental and emotional health. Essential oils stand out as flexible tools for fostering emotional resilience in our fast-paced and demanding lives as we continue to investigate the delicate relationship between aroma and mood. Including these fragrant jewels in everyday routines has the potential to improve emotional well-being and create a resilient attitude.

THE END